INNER LONGEVITY

The Science and Art of Living Well for Longer

Dr. VITA LONG

DEDICATION

Dedicated to my beautiful family

"The greatest wealth is health."

Virgil

CONTENTS

ACKNOWLEDGMENTS..i

Preface..ii

Chapter 1: Unlocking the Secrets of Longevity: Lessons from the world's longest-living people..........1

    1.1.   The Blue Zones...................................3

    1.2.   The Okinawans.................................5

    1.3.   The Sardinians.................................6

    1.4.   The Nicoyans....................................7

    1.5.   The Adventists.................................8

    1.6.   Lessons Learned.............................10

    1.7.   Key Takeaway................................11

Chapter 2: Understanding Aging: The latest discoveries and what they mean for your health.......12

    2.1. The Biology of Aging..........................13

    2.2. The Health Effects of Aging................15

    2.3. The Psychological Aspects of Aging.............16

    2.4. The Future of Aging...........................17

    2.5. Key Takeaways................................18

Chapter 3: The Anti-Aging Revolution: Separating fact from fiction...20

    3.1. The Science of Aging.........................21

    3.2. Common Anti-Aging Myths and

Misconceptions 23

3.3. The Ethics of Anti-Aging Research 26

3.4. Key Takeaways 29

Chapter 4: Fueling Your Body: The role of nutrition in longevity 31

4.1. The Science of Nutrition and Aging 32

4.2. Nutrients and Their Impact on Lifespan 33

4.3. Nutritional Strategies for Longevity 35

4.4. The Ethics of Nutrition and Aging 36

4.5. Conclusion 38

Chapter 5: Moving Towards Longevity: The importance of exercise and physical activity 40

5.1. Understanding the Science of Exercise and Longevity 41

5.2. The Types of Exercise and Their Benefits 42

5.3. Perform Aerobic Exercise: 42

a. Lifting Heavy Weights: 43

b. Exercises for Flexibility and Stability: 43

5.4. Creating an Individualized Workout Program to Promote Healthspan 44

5.5. Physical Exercise and Its Role in Everyday Life 46

5.6. Conclusion 48

Chapter 6: Enhancing Your Mind: Strategies for brain

health and longevity..49

6.1. Methods for Improving Brain Health and
Extending the Human Lifespan.............................51

a. Diet...51

b. Exercise 52

c. Sleep..52

6.2. Mental Stimulation and Social Engagement..53

a. Mental Stimulation 53

b. Social Engagement.............................53

6.3. Scientific Advances in Brain Health and
Longevity..54

a. Brain-Computer Interfaces 54

b. The neuroplasticity of the brain......................55

6.4. The Last Thoughts 56

7. The FINAL THOUGHTS 57

ACKNOWLEDGMENTS

I would like to express my deepest gratitude to my family for their unwavering support and encouragement throughout the writing of this book. Their love, patience, and understanding have been a constant source of inspiration and motivation.

PREFACE

Welcome to "Inner Longevity: The Science and Art of Living Well for Longer." This book will delve into the latest research and real-world advice for improving your health, preventing disease, and living a long, happy life. We all hope to enjoy a long and healthy life span since that is what it means to be human. But it's hard to know where to begin or who to trust when there's so much information and advice out there that contradicts itself. That's why I wrote this book: to give you a crash course in the science of longevity and give you actionable steps you can take to improve your personal health and longevity. The first three chapters of this book delve into the science of longevity, revealing the newest findings in the study of ageing, the techniques used by the world's longest-lived individuals, and the reality behind popular anti-aging nostrums. In rest of the three chapters, we'll look into specific methods for maintaining a healthy body and mind through things like diet, exercise, and mental stimulation.

CHAPTER 1: UNLOCKING THE SECRETS OF LONGEVITY: LESSONS FROM THE WORLD'S LONGEST-LIVING PEOPLE

The renowned philosopher Aristotle is credited with seeing, *"We are what we repeatedly do. Excellence, then, is not an act but a habit."*

The world's oldest people are living proof of this since they have perfected rituals and ways of life that extend their lives.

It's no secret that modern societies have the highest life expectancy rates in human history. Because of advances in medicine, technology, and better living circumstances, life expectancy has grown considerably during the last century. But what if I told you that there are regions of the world where living to be far over a hundred is the norm rather than the exception? These communities, known as "Blue Zones," are home to some of the world's longest-living individuals.

Here, we'll begin our investigation into the mysteries of longevity by speaking with some of the world's oldest individuals. We shall investigate the ways of life of centenarians from all over the world, from the quaint towns of Japan to the forested peaks of Ecuador.

People in the Blue Zones live longer and healthier lives than those in any other part of the world. Sardinia, Okinawa, Loma Linda, Nicoya, Costa Rica, and Ikaria, Greece are just some of the places in the world that fall under this category. Researchers have shown that these groups have many things in common, including ways of life, food, and social networks.

We'll go into what makes each of these groups, from the Blue Zones to the Seventh-Day Adventists, so successful at maintaining healthy, long lives. We may learn about grit, flexibility, and the value of finding one's niche in life from their experiences.

Consider the Loma Linda, California, congregation of the Seventh-day Adventist Church as an illustration. This group has gained notoriety for its members' commitment to a plant-based diet, rigors exercise regimen, and supportive social network. Taking time out of their hectic schedules to rest and recharge is equally important to them, as is tending to their spiritual health. These habits have been linked to longer and healthier lives, according to studies.

Okinawa, a Japanese island, provides yet another illustration. Vegetables, tofu, and seafood make up a large portion of the Okinawan diet. In addition, they engage in tai chi, a kind of martial arts known for improving both stability and mobility. The people of this area are also renowned for their close-knit communities, or "moai," in which members remain lifelong friends and support systems.

As a writer, I feel that learning the secrets of

longevity may educate us about how to live a rich and meaningful life, and is thus crucial to our own health and well-being. We can take cues from these groups on the value of regular exercise, nutritious food, and positive relationships.

The necessity of having a goal in life is emphasized, which is possibly the most valuable thing we can learn from these groups. The key to a long and happy life is finding meaning in what we do every day, whether that's through religion, family, or volunteer work.

So come with me as we explore the meaning of a life well-lived and the secrets to unleashing the power of our inner longevity. Lessons about how to live a long, healthy, and meaningful life can be gleaned from the experiences and habits of the world's longest-lived people.

1.1.   The Blue Zones

You can't ignore the idea of Blue Zones if you want to learn the secrets of longevity. People in some parts of the world not only outlive everyone else, but also enjoy better health overall. People in these areas tend to have high levels of life satisfaction, regular exercise, and a plant-based diet.

According to National Geographic and longevity researcher Dan Buettner, there are five distinct "Blue Zones" around the world, each with its own set of factors contributing to a high life expectancy.

Ikaria, Greece is home to the world's first Blue Zone. In this area, one-third of the population celebrates their 90th birthday, while dementia and cardiovascular disease are quite uncommon. The diet of beans, whole grains, and vegetables plays a large role in this. In addition, living in Ikaria is easygoing, so there's always time for friends, family, and leisure activities.

The men of Sardinia, Italy, the second Blue Zone, live exceptionally long lives. The island has the highest population of centenarians in the world, with one in every six men living to be over 100. Fruits, vegetables, and heart-healthy olive oil are staples in the Mediterranean diet that the people of Sardinia adhere to. Family values and multigenerational households are highly valued in this area.

Nicoya, Costa Rica, is home to the third Blue Zone, where residents enjoy a life expectancy that ranks in the top ten worldwide. The Nicoyans have a keen sense of direction and subsist on a diet of corn, beans, and tropical fruits. They also have robust social networks in the form of close-knit communities and large, nuclear families.

Loma Linda, California is home to a Seventh-Day Adventist community with a life expectancy that is ten years higher than the national average, making it the fourth Blue Zone. Many Adventists are avid hikers and cyclists because of the group's emphasis on a vegetarian diet and regular exercise. Longevity and happiness are also associated with the community's deep religious and civic commitments.

The highest life expectancy in the world is found in Okinawa, Japan, the fifth and last Blue Zone. Foods like sweet potatoes, soy products, and vegetables make up a large part of the Okinawans' plant-based diet. They also do little exercise like gardening and walking on a regular basis. Close family ties and a cultural emphasis on discovering one's "ikigai" (life's ultimate calling) contribute to Okinawans' robust feeling of community and purpose.

The habits and traditions that contribute to these Blue Zones' extraordinary lifespan are what set them apart. Looking at the lifestyles of these groups might teach us a lot about what it takes to live a long and happy life.

1.2.   The Okinawans

Okinawans, a native population of Japan's Ryukyu Islands, have been studied extensively because of their exceptionally high life expectancy. They have an average lifetime of nearly 90 years, making them one of the world's longest-living populations.

But what is it about their culture and way of life that permits them to live to such ripe old ages? The secret is in their nutrition and way of life, which they have perfected over generations of eco-friendly living.

Vegetables, whole grains, fish, and soy products are staples of the Okinawan diet. Miso and natto, two fermented foods high in beneficial bacteria, are staples in their diet. Okinawans tend to eat less meat, dairy, and processed foods than people in the West.

Yet, eating habits are simply one factor. The Okinawan way of life places a premium on having meaningful relationships, staying active, and having a clear sense of direction in one's life. Family and community are highly valued, and frequent opportunities arise throughout the day to engage with others. Moai, or a group of friends that stick together through thick and thin, is a common social institution in Okinawan society.

In Okinawa, exercise is an integral part of daily life. Traditional karate, for instance, is not just a method of self-defence but also of keeping fit and disciplined in mind and body. Okinawans are renowned for their agility and strength even as they age.

Ikigai, which means "a reason for being" in Okinawan, is a notion that helps Okinawans find meaning in their lives. Meaningful living is the result of paying attention to and acting on one's interests, skills, and values.

We can all learn a lot about how to live a longer, healthier, and more satisfying life by looking to the Okinawans for inspiration. The Okinawans serve as a useful reminder that a long and healthy life depends on more than simply good eating and regular exercise.

1.3.   The Sardinians

Sardinia, an Italian island, is home to a larger percentage of centenarians per population than any other of the world's five Blue Zones. Two major determinants in their lengthy life span are the quality of their nutrition and their social networks.

Vegetables, legumes, whole grains, and healthy fats like olive oil make up the bulk of the average Sardinian's diet. The typical food of these people is known as the "Mediterranean diet," and it has been linked to several health benefits, such as a lower risk of cardiovascular disease, diabetes, and Alzheimer's. The wine the Sardinians drink is full of antioxidants, and they drink it in moderation.

The Sardinian people are known for their excellent health and the closeness of their society. The Sardinian word "jentu," meaning "together," is fundamental to their culture and customs. The practice of eating together as a group has been shown to have health benefits, including lowered stress levels and increased immunity.

In addition to having a strong work ethic, Sardinians are also very active people who enjoy walking, gardening, and herding sheep throughout their life. Low-impact exercise like these helps seniors keep their fitness and independence for as long as possible.

The Sardinians have a tendency of eating lots of goat's milk and cheese, which is good for their bones because it contains calcium and vitamin D. Wild herbs are also a popular part of the Sardinian diet because of their high levels of antioxidants and other healthful elements.

Because of their healthy food, robust social networks, and active lifestyle, the people of Sardinia provide invaluable insights into the secrets of longevity. Their customs and routines can teach us how to live longer and healthier lives.

1.4.   The Nicoyans

The Nicoyan people are a rare subset of the Blue Zones, celebrated for their exceptional longevity and communal spirit. The Nicoya Peninsula of Costa Rica is home to an astounding number of centenarians and supercentenarians, giving the area one of the greatest life expectancies in the world.

The Nicoyan diet is said to be one reason why people live so long there. Beans, rice, corn, and tropical fruits are staples of the traditional Nicoyan diet. Eggs, dairy, and fish are also part of their diet, though in much smaller quantities. Reduce your chances of developing diabetes, heart disease, and cancer with this high-nutrient, high-antioxidant, high-fiber diet.

Longevity among Nicoyans, however, is not attributable primarily to their nutrition. A significant part of their culture is a focus on family and close friendships. Families in Nicoya frequently share housing, and residents place a premium on getting to know their neighbors. Positive effects on health have been linked to increased social connectedness and decreased stress.

Walks, gardens, and other sorts of manual labor are all part of the everyday routine for the Nicoyans. Their excellent health and lifespan can be attributed to their busy lifestyle, nutritious diet, and close-knit community.

The Nicoyan way of life emphasizes moderation in all things, from food to exercise to relationships. If we take cues from their lifestyle choices, we can enhance our own health and boost our chances of living a long and fruitful life for ourselves.

1.5.   The Adventists

Christian Seventh-Day Adventists, who number over 20 million globally, are another group designated as a Blue Zone. Many of their members live into their nineties and beyond, a feat made possible by their healthy way of life and food.

Many Adventists adhere to a healthy and active lifestyle by engaging in activities like frequent exercise and eating a plant-based diet. Adventists who adhere to a vegetarian or vegan diet have been demonstrated to have a lower risk of developing diabetes, heart disease, and cancer.

Adventists have a higher life expectancy than the general population for many reasons, including their devotion to God and healthy lifestyle habits. Sabbath observance, rest, and relaxation are promoted to help members cope with stress and improve their overall health. It has been established that the robust support network provided by Adventists' emphasis on spirituality and community contributes to their general health and lifespan.

Adventists place a premium on eating whole foods, which is one of many habits that has been shown to increase life expectancy. Adventists often eat unprocessed meals such as fresh produce, whole grains, and nuts instead of packaged and processed goods. They also stay away from unhealthy substances like caffeine, alcohol, and tobacco.

The Japanese proverb hara hachi bu, which translates to "eat until you're 80% full," is another factor in Adventists' extended life expectancy. Adventists can avoid obesity and other health issues by following this principle and exercising self-control at mealtimes.

Adventists also place a high value on physical activity and methods of stress reduction, such as yoga and meditation. Both the body and the mind benefit from these routines, making them excellent ways to extend your life.

The Seventh-day Adventist community is an exceptional case study of the positive effects of a combination of secular and religious behaviors on longevity. To live a full and fruitful life, one must take care of one's body, mind, and spirit, and they show us the way.

1.6.   Lessons Learned

We have learned a great deal about the secrets of longevity from studying the habits, diets, and relationships of the world's longest-living people. These groups, from the Okinawans to the Seventh-Day Adventists, have taught us a great deal that we may incorporate into our own lives.

The significance of family and friends networks stands out as a universal factor in all Blue Zones. The Nicoyans, the Sardinians, and the Adventists all place a premium on family and community, and all three groups' members live longer and healthier as a result of their strong social networks.

A balanced and nutritious diet is very important if you want to live a long and healthy life. Communities all across the world, from the Okinawans and Adventists to the Sardinians and their traditional Mediterranean diet, have taught us the value of eating complete, unprocessed foods that are high in minerals and antioxidants.

Yet how we eat is just as important as what we eat. Sardinians adopt moderation and portion management, but Okinawans adhere to the concept of Hara Hachi Bu, which implies eating until you are 80% satisfied. By incorporating these practices and listening to our internal cues, we may control our appetite, improve our digestion, and enhance our general well-being.

Last but not least, studies have linked a healthy feeling of meaning and purpose to a longer life span. While Adventists place a premium on religious observances and volunteer work, Nicoyans place a similar emphasis on passing down knowledge and customs from generation to generation. To live a longer, healthier life, it is important to discover and pursue our individual hobbies and ambitions.

The experiences of the world's longest-lived individuals have much to teach us. We can improve our chances of living long, happy lives by putting our focus on our relationships, eating well, and discovering what gives our life value. Hence, let's take these insights to heart and activate our inner fountain of youth.

1.7.   Key Takeaway

I've always been curious about the science behind agelessness. There are some routines and routines that can help us live longer, healthier lives, as we have seen from the Blue Zones and the anecdotes of its people. The Okinawans with their plant-based diets have much to teach the Nicoyans about the importance of community, and vice versa.

As we get to the end of this chapter, I'd want to stress the significance of learning these secrets of long life. Doing so can help us take charge of our health and happiness, leading to a richer, fuller life overall.

We'll learn more about heredity's impact on lifespan in the future chapter. A person's lifespan can be affected not just by their genes, but also by their surroundings and their decisions in how they live. If you want to live a longer, healthier life, then come with me as we explore the science of longevity.

CHAPTER 2: UNDERSTANDING AGING: THE LATEST DISCOVERIES AND WHAT THEY MEAN FOR YOUR HEALTH

In the quiet of the morning, when the light peeks over the horizon and the birds begin to sing, it is hard not to think about the bigger questions of life. Time is a precious commodity that each of us is given at birth, yet it seems that our time here on Earth is brief, and before we realize it, old age sets in and our bodies begin to deteriorate. But imagine if we could unlock the mysteries of aging and apply that knowledge to live longer healthier, and happier lives.

In this section, we take a trip into the domain of science and discovery to examine the most recent findings on aging and its effects on health. By delving into these questions, we can gain a better understanding of the causes of aging, the elements that contribute to its development, and the most recent findings in the field of anti-aging medicine.

We will explore the science of aging from the

molecular to the societal levels, looking at how our genes, lifestyle choices and the environment influence our health as we become older. By conducting this study, we can learn more about ways to delay aging and extend our healthy life span.

Thus, my reader, I ask you to join me on this voyage of discovery as we learn to embrace life with vitality and vigor despite the inevitable passage of time.

2.1. The Biology of Aging

Here, we explore the complex biological mechanisms behind aging and attempt to unravel some of its secrets. Simply said, aging is an inevitable process of aging that affects every living thing. Yet, aging is not a simple process and is driven by a complicated set of systems, the details of which remain a mystery to us.

For a long time, researchers have been trying to figure out the biology behind aging. The abundance of competing hypotheses that attempt to explain aging and its causes presents a significant obstacle to research. There are many different hypotheses about what causes aging, from the damage accumulation hypothesis, which holds that the accumulation of molecular damage in our cells is to blame, to the programmed theory, which holds that aging is a natural consequence of our genetic programming.

Recent years, however, have seen major breakthroughs in the study of aging, providing new insight into this nuanced process. The significance of cellular senescence, in which cells cease dividing and enter a latent state, has been one of the most fascinating findings. Scientists are looking into targeting senescent cells as a possible anti-aging strategy because it is believed that this process contributes to aging and age-related disorders.

The significance of DNA damage in the aging process is another major finding. Constant exposure to environmental conditions, such as radiation and chemicals, puts our DNA at risk of mutations and other defects. The accumulation of this damage over time causes cellular malfunction and ultimately aging. Scientists are currently looking at potential solutions to reverse this damage and forestall or postpone the onset of age-related disorders.

New insights into the systems that contribute to the aging process are being uncovered as the study of aging develops. New insights from the study of aging have revealed how cellular senescence and DNA damage contribute to the aging process.

Over time, cells lose their ability to proliferate and function normally, a phenomenon known as cellular senescence. Cellular senescence has been linked to the buildup of damaged cells in the body and, by extension, the aging process. These compromised cells can set off detrimental processes that hasten to age, such as chronic inflammation.

DNA damage has been the focus of several recent investigations on the aging process as well as cellular senescence. Exposure to environmental chemicals, radiation, and other factors can cause DNA damage, which can build up over time. Its destruction can trigger gene alterations and promote the onset of age-related illnesses like cancer.

Researchers are discovering new opportunities for anti-aging medicines as they get a deeper grasp of the fundamental systems that contribute to the aging process. Others are working on gene therapies to repair

DNA damage and prevent mutations, while others are investigating the potential of medications that might specifically target and kill senescent cells.

Our newfound knowledge of aging and the promising potential of potential anti-aging medicines are the results of these and similar findings. Perhaps we might enhance our health and live longer if we attack the causes of aging at their biological roots. Recent findings in the study of aging offer hope for a deeper comprehension of the aging process and the creation of effective novel therapies to support active, healthy old age.

2.2. The Health Effects of Aging

The danger of getting diseases like cardiovascular disease, Alzheimer's, and osteoporosis rises as people get older because of the changes that occur in their bodies. For instance, as we age, our arteries may stiffen, making it more difficult for blood to flow as it should. This can increase the risk of cardiovascular disease. The risk of osteoporosis may also rise if our bones grow more brittle and break easily.

Alterations to the immune system are another major consequence of getting older. Our ability to recognize and fight off germs declines with age, making us more vulnerable to infectious diseases. Chronic inflammation, which can be exacerbated by this, has been related to many different diseases and disorders, including heart disease, diabetes, and even some forms of cancer.

But new studies reveal that we may lessen the negative consequences of aging on our bodies in important ways. Exercising frequently, for instance, has been linked to better cardiovascular health and a lower risk of chronic disease. Overall health can be supported by eating a diet high in fruits, vegetables, and whole grains.

Vitamin and mineral supplements have also demonstrated potential for promoting healthy aging. Vitamin D supplementation, for instance, has been demonstrated to increase bone density and decrease fracture risk in elderly people.

By being aware of the most common negative health outcomes associated with aging and the most recent findings on how to counteract these outcomes, we may take preventative measures to ensure our continued health and happiness as we age.

2.3. The Psychological Aspects of Aging

Aging can have profound implications on a person's mental and emotional health as well as their physical health. It can be difficult to have a sense of purpose in life and we may suffer with emotions of isolation, despair, and worry as we become older.

These mental obstacles can have a major effect on our quality of life as we get older, so it's important to recognize them and work to overcome them. Loneliness and isolation are as damaging to our health as smoking and being overweight, according to research. That's why it's so important to stay in touch with loved ones and be involved in your neighborhood.

Having a goal in life and knowing why we're here can improve our health and happiness. Having a sense of meaning in life has been linked to improved physical and mental health in later life. Feeling fulfilled and having a purpose in life can be aided by engaging in meaningful activities such as volunteering or pursuing hobbies.

Meditation and other mindfulness activities have gained favor in recent years as proven strategies for improving the emotional well-being of the elderly. Mindfulness meditation has been demonstrated to promote mental health and decrease stress and despair. Mindfulness training has been shown to have positive effects on both self-awareness and emotional regulation, both of which can be especially useful for dealing with the difficulties that come with aging.

In conclusion, the mental effects of aging are equally as significant as the physical ones. The quality of our lives as we get older can be enhanced by coping with emotional and psychological difficulties, staying connected with others, and finding meaningful work to do. Mindfulness techniques not only help us age gracefully but also improve our overall mental health.

2.4. The Future of Aging

We are on the threshold of some genuinely extraordinary discoveries as we learn more about the complexities of aging. New research techniques and technologies are opening up exciting opportunities in the study of aging.

Regenerative medicine is one such technique, with the goal of mending malfunctioning bodily organs and tissues. Stem cell research, gene therapy, and other promising new methods for repairing damaged tissue and slowing the aging process are all being investigated.

The study of artificial intelligence (AI) is also relevant to the study of aging. Artificial intelligence

(AI) has the potential to improve illness prevention and management due to its capacity to analyze large volumes of data and discover trends. Scientists are working on AI-driven systems for remote patient monitoring, disease prognosis, and potentially individualized treatment.

The way we view and deal with aging might change as these technologies go further. Prevention of age-related diseases may be preferable to treating their symptoms. Personalized medicine, which takes into account an individual's specific genetic composition and health care requirements, may also gain prominence.

It is evident that we are on the verge of a new era in the study of aging, even if there is still much to be discovered about the aging process. Investing in new technologies and expanding our understanding of the aging process could lead to breakthroughs in health and lifespan promotion.

2.5. Key Takeaways

This chapter has shown us that aging is a multifaceted process that has far-reaching consequences. Knowing how the aging process works from the inside out, from the underlying biological mechanics to the potential mental health issues that can arise, is essential to age effectively.

We have examined how recent findings in the study of aging, such as the significance of DNA damage and cellular senescence, are altering our conception of aging and the potential for anti-aging therapies.

We've also covered the newest studies on how to lessen the negative impacts of aging on our health through things like exercise, diet, and supplements for things like cardiovascular disease, Alzheimer's, and osteoporosis.

We have also highlighted the significance of keeping up social relationships and a sense of purpose as we age, as well as the emotional and psychological difficulties that might occur with aging, such as loneliness and depression.

We have considered the potential implications of future developments in the field of aging research, such as regenerative medicine and the application of artificial intelligence to the prevention and management of the disease.

Keeping up with the latest findings in the study of aging is crucial to our health and well-being as we age. In the following chapter, we will go more deeply into the issue of disease prevention and management, investigating the most up-to-date strategies and approaches for maintaining physical and mental health throughout the aging process.

CHAPTER 3: THE ANTI-AGING REVOLUTION: SEPARATING FACT FROM FICTION

At one time, many believed that the Fountain of Youth was nothing more than a fantastical urban legend. But, as science and medicine have advanced, the prospect of anti-aging medicines has moved beyond the realm of science fiction. The search for the fountain of youth has become a multibillion-dollar industry.

One negative aspect of the expanding market for anti-aging therapies is the proliferation of unsubstantiated claims. There are many unreliable sources in the field of anti-aging studies, from "snake oil" marketers to social media influencers selling the newest "wonder" remedy.

Aristotle stated, "*The aim of life is to live it, to taste experience to the fullest, to reach out enthusiastically and without fear for a fresh and deeper experience,*" and what could be more enriching than the prospect of stopping or at least slowing down the aging process? For millennia, humanity has tried to find a way to stay young forever.

Now, thanks to scientific progress, that dream is within reach. Yet like with any promising new area, others would take advantage of the public's eagerness to get on the bandwagon. In this chapter, we will sort through the myths and bogus research surrounding anti-aging therapies to get to the bottom of things. Join us as we investigate the claims and counterclaims surrounding the anti-aging movement and uncover its true potential.

This section will help with that. We will investigate recent scientific findings and sort facts from fiction. It's time to sort through the hype around anti-aging therapies and get to the bottom of what works. So, unwind, because we are about to explore the Anti-Aging Revolution.

3.1. The Science of Aging

Before delving into anti-aging practices, it is important to get a firm grasp on how aging works from a scientific perspective. As we get older, our bodies and minds change due to the natural process of aging. Although becoming older is inevitable, it frequently comes with age-related disorders like cancer, heart disease, and Alzheimer's that can have a devastating effect on our quality of life.

Recent years have seen a rise in the popularity of anti-aging treatments that aim to prevent or delay the onset of age-related disorders. Our current understanding of the aging process is limited, however, and it is crucial to remember that the science of aging is still in its infancy.

While there have been encouraging developments in anti-aging research, such as the activation of telomerase and the use of senolytics to target senescent cells, much remains unknown. Anti-aging treatments are popular, but we need to proceed with caution because of the prevalence of pseudo-science and false information around them.

Therefore, it is crucial to separate reality from fantasy in anti-aging studies. In what follows, we'll take a closer look at the most recent findings in the field of anti-aging science and determine which treatments have the potential to improve our health and add years to our lives, and which are a waste of time and money.

Age-related disorders are conditions that are more likely to manifest as we become older, although aging is a normal process that impacts all organisms. Heart disease, cancer, Alzheimer's disease, and osteoporosis are just a few of the age-related illnesses that plague the elderly. Age-related disorders share some biological processes with aging, although they are not the same.

Most current anti-aging therapies aim to slow down or even reverse the body's natural aging processes by targeting things like oxidative stress and inflammation. Nevertheless, these therapies do not exist in a vacuum. In animal models, calorie restriction and exercise have been found to slow aging; however, the advantages of these practices on people are still being researched. Similarly, scant data is supporting the efficacy of other anti-aging therapies, including some nutritional supplements.

Knowing the facts about aging and age-related disorders, as well as the limitations of current anti-aging treatments, is crucial for determining what is true and what is not in the field of anti-aging research.

Current anti-aging treatments have their drawbacks,

but the field of anti-aging research is making remarkable strides. Gene therapy, stem cell studies, and epigenetic manipulation are just some of the new approaches to anti-aging that scientists are investigating. The future of effective anti-aging medicines may lie with these methods, which have shown promise in animal research and preliminary human trials.

The use of Artificial Intelligence (AI) and Machine Learning (ML) in the study of aging and the discovery of novel therapeutic targets is another exciting field of study. These tools could significantly advance anti-aging studies by facilitating the analysis of massive datasets and the identification of previously unknown relationships and patterns.

In conclusion, anti-aging science is a dynamic and intricate field. A deeper understanding of the biology of aging and the development of safe and effective anti-aging medicines has the potential to dramatically enhance the health span and quality of life for aging populations, but there is no silver bullet for stopping or reversing the aging process. By distinguishing fact from fiction and putting an emphasis on evidence-based research, we may contribute to the development of the next generation of anti-aging medicines that are secure, efficient, and really revolutionary.

3.2. Common Anti-Aging Myths and Misconceptions

In this section, we'll debunk some of the most pervasive myths regarding anti-aging treatments. There is a lot of disinformation and pseudo-science out there, despite the increased interest in the topic. The truth of anti-aging can be uncovered by evaluating claims against scientific evidence.

The idea that anti-aging supplements may reverse time passing is a widely held but false concept. No miracle drug can stop or reverse aging, while certain nutrients can aid in general health and well-being. Some research suggests that taking too much of various supplements can be dangerous.

The significance of telomeres in the aging process is another widely held false belief. The chromosomal endcaps called telomeres have been related to cellular degeneration. Yet, it is highly improbable that taking a telomerase supplement or undertaking telomere therapy on their own would have a major impact on the aging process as a whole. Although telomeres are a vital part of the anti-aging jigsaw, they are not the only factor to consider.

These and other anti-aging misconceptions need to be dispelled so that we may begin to concentrate on the therapies and tactics that truly work. There are numerous tried-and-true methods for keeping our health and vitality as we age, including exercise, diet, skincare, and mindfulness.

Vitamin and mineral supplements, in particular, have gained popularity among those who hope to delay or even reverse the effects of aging. While it's true that some vitamins and minerals are necessary for optimum health, there's not much proof that taking mega-doses of these nutrients may slow down the aging process.

The idea that telomeres, the caps at the ends of our chromosomes, are the secret to delaying aging is another popular misconception. Although telomeres are involved in the aging process, studies have demonstrated that the mechanisms by which telomeres contribute to aging are complex and not fully understood.

When it comes to anti-aging therapies, truth from fiction is essential. There are many intriguing research avenues, but we still have a long way to go in understanding the aging process and how to slow it. It's important to think critically about anti-aging treatments and get medical advice before trying something new.

It is crucial to keep up with the most recent findings and promising approaches in the field of anti-aging research. The potential of various treatments, such as senolytics and NAD+ precursors, to increase longevity and improve health span is now the subject of a large number of studies.

So, we must approach these interventions critically and take into account their possible downsides. Extending life expectancy with calorie restriction, for instance, has shown promise in animal research but may be difficult to maintain in humans and could have detrimental side effects.

Hormone replacement therapy is another anti-aging treatment that has been debunked by science because it has been linked to an increased risk of cancer and other health problems. Before starting any anti-aging treatment, it's important to think about the pros and cons.

As science develops, new and creative approaches with fresh potential for extending healthy longevity are expected to be developed. It's crucial to be educated and know the difference between fact and fiction in order to make the best decisions for our health and welfare.

There may be benefits to certain therapies, but there may also be drawbacks that need to be considered. Several animal models have proven that calorie restriction can extend their lives, however, this may not be an option for people. Hormone replacement treatment has been associated with an increase in the risk of certain malignancies while also helping to lessen some of the negative effects of aging.

The area of anti-aging research is quickly growing, but there is still much to learn about the aging process and prospective cures. It's important to consider anti-aging therapies cautiously, distinguishing reality from fiction, and assessing the benefits and drawbacks of different operations. By doing this, we can make better decisions for our long-term health and pleasure.

Despite the fact that anti-aging medicines and interventions may hold enormous promise for improving our health and extending our lives, it is important to approach them with care and skepticism. Our capacity to stay up with the most recent scientific developments and distinguish fact from fiction will determine our health and well-being as we age. The relationship between what you eat and how you feel as you get older will be covered in detail in the next chapter.

3.3. The Ethics of Anti-Aging Research

We must consider the moral implications of these prospective therapies as we explore the promising directions of anti-aging technology. A major reason for concern is the potential for prejudice and unfairness in the allocation of treatments. Anti-aging treatments might end up becoming a luxury available only to the wealthy, further separating society into those who can afford to pay to live longer and those who cannot. This may have far-reaching effects on society and make current disparities worse.

The possibility of unforeseen outcomes also raises ethical concerns. Anti-aging procedures have the potential to increase human life expectancy, but this development could have far-reaching consequences for our planet, our economy, and our society. We need to watch out that our efforts to live longer do not come at the expense of the next generation or the world.

Ethical and responsible anti-aging research is essential for addressing these issues. This involves thinking about the bigger picture and making sure that everyone, regardless of socioeconomic status, has access to the therapies they need. By approaching anti-aging research with care and caution, we can ensure that its benefits are shared by all and that inequalities are not exacerbated in the future.

There are serious moral concerns that must be addressed about the search for anti-aging therapies. The potential for bias and disparity in the distribution of these treatments is a major cause for alarm. Inequalities may worsen or emerge if only the wealthy or privileged have access to medicines that extend life or restore youthfulness.

Using animals in anti-aging studies raises similar moral concerns. Some people think it's unethical and pointless to conduct research on animals, although it's helped humans learn a lot about things like how the body ages and how diseases develop. The potential advantages of studying against the costs of using animals in that research must be carefully weighed.

Finally, anti-aging studies and therapies need to be conducted reasonably and equitably. This includes providing everyone with the same chances to take part in research and get treatment, as well as access to information and services related to aging. This also includes not taking advantage of the elderly or the disabled in your quest for anti-aging treatments.

To guarantee that our efforts to extend and improve human lifespan are responsible, equitable, and sustainable, we must keep these ethical concerns in mind as the area of anti-aging research develops further. This is the only way to ensure that people from all walks of life, regardless of their socioeconomic situation, may reap the advantages of anti-aging research.

There is also the worry that anti-aging medicine will foster prejudice and inequity. There may be a growing gap between people who can and cannot afford these medicines as they become more generally offered. Since these therapies may be prohibitively expensive and hence only accessible to those with greater financial means, it is crucial to investigate how to ensure that they are made available on an equitable basis.

Anti-aging research must be undertaken responsibly and equitably if these ethical problems are to be addressed. This involves making sure that the benefits and hazards of medicines are thoroughly studied before they are made available to the public and that clinical studies are undertaken with a wide range of participants. The long-term impacts of anti-aging treatments, on both people and on society as a whole, must also be taken into account.

In conclusion, anti-aging research has the potential to greatly benefit human health and longevity into old age, but it must be approached with caution and the two extremes must be distinguished. We may move closer to a future where we can all age gracefully and healthily by comprehending the current status of anti-aging research, dispelling prevalent myths and misconceptions, and analyzing the ethical considerations surrounding these treatments.

3.4. Key Takeaways

As we wrap up our look at the anti-aging revolution, it's clear that there's still a lot we don't know. There are many myths and pseudo-sciences about anti-aging treatments, but there are also potential strategies being explored now that may help us live healthier for longer in the future. Yet, we should approach these treatments critically and with an educated grasp of their advantages and disadvantages.

The goal of immortality should not be encouraged, and everyone should have equal access to anti-aging medicines, therefore it's important to think about the moral implications of this field of study. inequality or discrimination. By considering both the scientific and ethical aspects of anti-aging research, we can work towards responsible and sustainable approaches to extending the human health span.

In the next chapter, we will explore the complex relationship between aging and disease, investigating how our understanding of aging can inform disease prevention and treatment. We will also examine the latest research on age-related diseases such as

Alzheimer's and cancer and the potential for interventions that could help us live healthier and more fulfilling lives as we age.

It is critical to understand that anti-aging science is still in its infancy and that much remains to be learned. Although there are continuing research and potential initiatives in the sector, there is also a lot of false information that must be disproven. Before attempting any new therapies, people should speak with healthcare specialists and adopt a critical and educated viewpoint when approaching anti-aging treatments.

The research and use of anti-aging medicines must also take ethical issues into account. Responsible and equitable methods of anti-aging research and therapy are required to address the possibility of discrimination and disparity in access to therapies.

We will go into more detail on the relationship between aging and mental health in the next chapter. We will review the most recent studies on preserving mental health in older persons as well as the emotional and psychological difficulties that come with aging. So come along with us as we venture more into the interesting field of aging research.

CHAPTER 4: FUELING YOUR BODY: THE ROLE OF NUTRITION IN LONGEVITY

"Let food be thy medicine and medicine be thy food." These same words were stated by Hippocrates, an ancient Greek physician, and they still hold true today. He said them about two thousand years ago, yet they still hold true today. Our health is greatly influenced by the quality of the food we consume, and as we age, this becomes increasingly important. This chapter will teach us about the foods and eating habits that are associated with healthy aging as well as the relationship between the two. But before we get into the specifics, it's important to consider how nutrition affects aging and why eating properly is so crucial.

Our dietary requirements shift as we become older, making it even more crucial that we eat healthily to sustain our health and vitality. Nonetheless, many people have trouble sticking to healthy eating habits as they age, opting instead for diets high in saturated fat, sugar, and processed foods.

Key nutrients and dietary patterns linked to

longevity will be discussed in this chapter, along with their role in fostering good aging. The detrimental effects of inadequate nutrition on health and happiness will be analyzed, and methods for enhancing one's diet to promote healthy aging will be discussed.

The goal of this chapter is to equip readers with the knowledge and skills necessary to incorporate healthy eating habits into their daily lives, as well as an appreciation for the role nutrition plays in fostering healthy aging.

4.1. The Science of Nutrition and Aging

It has been theorized that the Elves' nutrition was a major factor in their legendary lifespans in Middle-earth. Modern science has demonstrated that our nutrition has a big impact on our health and the aging process, much as the Elves were mindful of what they ate.

The links between what we eat and how we age will be investigated in this chapter as we delve into the science of nutrition and aging. We will explore how inadequate nutrition might hasten the aging process and review the fundamentals of nutrition and its effect on health. We'll also talk about the ways in which eating right helps stave off degenerative diseases like diabetes, heart disease, and cancer as we become older.

The more we learn about the connection between food and longevity, the better decisions we may make to improve our health and quality of life. Let's dive headfirst into the science of food and longevity.

Cellular function and metabolic rate both deteriorate with age. Nutrient deficiencies and chronic diseases like heart disease, diabetes, and osteoporosis result when our bodies have a harder time absorbing and using the food we eat. There is still a lot to learn about the particular mechanisms by which nutrition affects aging, as its effects are multifaceted and complex. But, studies have proved over and over that eating well and doing enough exercise is crucial for aging well and warding off age-related disorders.

However, nutritional deficiencies might hasten the aging process. In particular, eating a lot of processed meals, refined carbohydrates, and bad fats can increase inflammation, oxidative stress, and tissue damage. These negative consequences may hasten aging and the progression of chronic diseases. Fruits, vegetables, whole grains, lean proteins, and healthy fats, on the other hand, can give the body the nutrients it needs to perform at its peak and support healthy aging when eaten as part of a diet that is otherwise high in processed foods.

To promote healthy aging and reduce the risk of age-related disorders, knowledge of the science of nutrition and aging is essential. In what follows, we'll take a closer look at the foods and eating habits that should be avoided, as well as the nutrients and dietary patterns that have been related to healthy aging and long life.

4.2. Nutrients and Their Impact on Lifespan

The old adage goes something like, "You are what you eat." The importance of proper nutrition to our well-being increases with age. Here, we'll talk about the nutrients seniors can't live without and how different diets affect how long they live.

To begin with, maintaining a healthy weight by eating a well-rounded diet rich in all the nutrients you need as you become older is crucial. Antioxidants, minerals, and vitamins are all important for warding off age-related disorders and staying healthy in general. Vitamin D is essential for strong bones, and vitamin C helps the body fight off free radicals and maintain a healthy immune system.

However, fad diets or severe diets that cut out entire food groups can be hazardous to human health and should be avoided at all costs. Finding a diet that is both healthy and sustainable is the key, as is limiting the intake of saturated fats, added sugars, and processed foods.

Many studies have investigated whether certain diets specifically increase lifespan. A diet rich in whole grains, fruits, vegetables, legumes, and healthy fats like olive oil has been demonstrated to lower the risk of cardiovascular disease and increase life expectancy. Lower incidences of cancer, heart disease, and diabetes have also been associated with plant-based diets.

Keep in mind that what works for one individual may not work for another when it comes to their nutritional demands. To make sure you're getting what you need for a long, healthy life, it's best to talk to a doctor or dietician.

This highlights the importance of proper nutrition in supporting good aging and a long life span. Extreme or fad diets should be avoided in favor of a balanced diet that contains all of the necessary nutrients. While some people may benefit more from plant-based or Mediterranean diets, others may not.

4.3. Nutritional Strategies for Longevity

As we delve more into the connection between food and health span, it's crucial to talk about ways to get people to adopt diets that will help them live longer and better. Mindful eating is one method in this category since it encourages one to be present when eating and to focus on one's senses. When we eat more slowly and mindfully, we take more pleasure from our food and are less likely to overeat.

Healthy eating and longevity can be promoted in other ways as well, for as through the practice of meal planning. Meal preparation in advance helps us acquire the variety of nutrients we need while avoiding unhealthy, impulsive choices. Those who are short on time or who must adhere to tight diets may benefit greatly from this.

It's wise to proceed with caution when using dietary supplements. Certain supplements may be helpful, while others may do more damage than good. If you are over 65 and have any preexisting health concerns, you should talk to your doctor before using any dietary supplements.

The potential for tailor-made diets made possible by innovations and dietary trends is enticing. For instance, genetic testing can reveal an individual's ancestry, which can be used to create a diet and supplement program that works for that person specifically. Further study is needed to properly understand the effects of these technologies on nutrition and aging, so we should approach them with care and skepticism.

New technology may significantly alter how we think about food and aging. Genetic testing is one such method, as it can give people unique insights into how their DNA affects their dietary preferences and vulnerability to disease.

Mobile apps and wearable gadgets that monitor dietary consumption, physical activity, and other health indicators have also been developed thanks to developments in digital health technology. Using these resources, people may keep tabs on their food and health and make better decisions about what works best for them.

Microbiome analysis as a tool for creating nutritional guidelines is another area of cutting-edge research. The bacteria that live in the human digestive tract, known as the gut microbiome, have a significant impact on the body's ability to absorb nutrients. Nutritionists and other medical experts can better advise their patients on how to eat to promote healthy aging by evaluating their microbiomes.

Maintaining a balanced and diverse diet, while also being attentive to the foods we eat and how they affect our health, is the key to supporting proper nutrition and longevity. A critical and well-informed approach to nutrition allows us to make decisions that support good aging and a longer, more rewarding life.

4.4. The Ethics of Nutrition and Aging

There are serious moral questions raised by the correlation between diet and longevity that must be addressed. Access to healthful meals is a fundamental ethical concern because it is a huge challenge for many people, especially those living in low-income areas or food deserts. Poor nutrition has been linked to an accelerated aging process, and it can be challenging to obtain economical and good food options in these places.

There is also the moral need to spread information about good eating practices, which is especially important in underserved areas. This is especially relevant for the elderly, who may have been exposed to a variety of cuisines and ways of life during their lifetimes. Healthy aging is facilitated by older persons making well-informed dietary choices, which can be facilitated through education.

Access to healthy food options, nutritional education, and cultural sensitivity are all essential components of responsible and equitable approaches to nutrition and aging. By addressing these issues, we can help everyone, regardless of their economic or cultural background, live as long and healthy a life as possible.

The availability of nutritious foods and the prevention of hunger are two examples of ethical concerns related to aging and nutrition. Food insecurity is a serious problem in many parts of the country, especially in low-income neighborhoods. This may contribute to a rise in diet-related health problems and exacerbate existing inequalities in health. Policymakers and communities must endeavor to ensure that all people, regardless of income or geography, have ready access to affordable, nutritious food.

The promotion of potentially harmful or unproven nutritional practices should be avoided, and evidence-based interventions should take precedence, to take a responsible and equitable approach. In addition, everyone should be able to afford nutritional interventions, not only the wealthy few who can afford to buy pricey supplements or pay personal nutritionists. Nutritional education and literacy should also be encouraged to equip people to make educated decisions about their meals and encourage good eating habits that will last a lifetime.

The benefits of exercise and other forms of physical activity on healthy aging will be discussed in the following chapter. We will examine the research on exercise's positive effects, talk about the difficulties of sustaining an active lifestyle, and present doable solutions for making exercise a regular part of your routine.

4.5. Conclusion

Let food be thy medicine and medicine be thy food, as Hippocrates once said. In this chapter, we explored the importance of diet in fostering longevity and quality of life as we age. We have discussed the research on nutrition and aging, the nutrients that are most important for maintaining health as we get older, and some of the nutritional approaches that can help you age well. We've looked at why it's important to have a responsible, fair approach to nutrition and aging, and what ethical concerns arise from dietary therapies for the elderly.

It's obvious that eating well is about more than just filling bellies and appeasing taste sensations; it's also about keeping us healthy and alive for as long as possible. To age healthily and avoid age-related ailments, one must take a well-rounded and conscientious approach to their diet. The quality of our lives as we age is directly related to the decisions we make about what and how much to eat.

In the following chapter, we will continue our investigation into aging by focusing on the benefits of exercise and physical activity. We will discuss the research on exercise and aging, the positive effects of exercise as we become older, and the many ways in which we may work exercise into our busy schedules. Come along with us as we continue our quest toward successful aging.

CHAPTER 5: MOVING TOWARDS LONGEVITY: THE IMPORTANCE OF EXERCISE AND PHYSICAL ACTIVITY

John Steinbeck's words, *"Adopt the pace of nature: her secret is patience,"* capture the essence of our existence. Our bodies were made to move, to embrace the natural rhythms of life. Yet in the modern world, we find ourselves trapped in sedentary lifestyles, glued to screens, and isolated from the natural world.

But there is hope: exercise and physical activity have been shown to help us not only live longer but live better. It is commonly recognized that regular physical activity and exercise have many positive health effects, such as better heart health, stronger bones, a decreased chance of developing chronic illnesses, and improved mental health.

In this chapter, we'll discover why physical activity and exercise are so important for maintaining a long and healthy life, as well as the most recent research on the health benefits of exercise and practical advice for fitting it into our busy lives. So take it easy, my reader, and follow me on this quest for a longer, better, and more fruitful life.

5.1. Understanding the Science of Exercise and Longevity

Regular exercise has been found to enhance our immune systems, increase our mental and emotional well-being, improve our cardiovascular health, lessen our risk of acquiring chronic illnesses, and even reverse the cellular aging process in addition to keeping us physically fit.

Several studies have shown the advantages of regular exercise for cardiovascular health. For instance, research indicated that those who frequently engaged in moderate to vigorous physical exercise had a decreased chance of getting heart disease than those who were sedentary. The study was published in the journal Circulation.

In a study that was published in the Journal of Clinical Oncology, researchers discovered a relationship between exercise and a reduced risk of breast cancer death and recurrence. Moreover, it has been shown that regular exercise increases bone density, lowering the incidence of fractures in older persons.

Frontiers in Aging Neuroscience research found a link between regular exercise and improved cognitive function in older people. Exercise has also been shown to improve mood by reducing the signs of melancholy and anxiety.

Another system that might gain from exercise is the immune system. Regular physical exercise has been associated in studies to improve immune function and reduced inflammation, both of which help prevent chronic illnesses and infections and reduce the chance of developing autoimmune disorders.

Last but not least, new research indicates that exercise may be able to delay cellular aging. High-intensity interval training (HIIT) increased mitochondrial function in older persons, according to research published in the journal Cell Metabolism. Mitochondria are essential for cellular health and energy synthesis.

The conclusion drawn from scientific research is that regular exercise and physical activity may significantly increase our lifespan. Exercise is a powerful tool for supporting a long and healthy life since it promotes immune system function, improves cardiovascular health, lowers the risk of chronic illnesses, improves mental and cognitive health, and slows cellular aging.

5.2. The Types of Exercise and Their Benefits

The three main forms of exercise and how they may improve your health and lengthen your life are discussed here. Not all forms of exercise have the same positive effects on lifespan, but they all go beyond just jogging on a treadmill or lifting weights.

5.3. Perform Aerobic Exercise:

Aerobic exercise, also known as cardiovascular exercise, lowers the risk of mortality from any cause by as much as 30 percent in people who regularly partake in activities like running, cycling, and swimming.

Regular aerobic exercise has been found to help reduce stress, anxiety, and depression, improve heart and lung function, lower the risk of chronic diseases like diabetes and high blood pressure, and increase overall health and longevity.

a. Lifting Heavy Weights:

Resistance training, also called strength or weight training, is a type of exercise in which weights or resistance bands are used to strengthen the muscles. This type of exercise is important for maintaining muscle mass and bone density as we age, which can help prevent falls and fractures.

b. Exercises for Flexibility and Stability:

A study published in the journal Age and Aging found that frequent flexibility and balance training can help minimize the risk of falls and enhance the overall quality of life in older persons because of the positive effects on mobility and stability.

Aim for at least 150 minutes of moderate aerobic activity, 75 minutes of strenuous aerobic exercise, and two days of resistance training each week, in addition to regular flexibility and balance training, for the benefits mentioned above and to avoid boredom and stay motivated.

Whether you enjoy running, doing weights, or practicing yoga, including all three in your program will ensure that you reap the greatest longevity advantages while also improving your quality of life.

Aerobic exercise, also known as cardio, involves activities that increase the heart rate and breathing, such as jogging, cycling, or swimming, and has been shown to have numerous benefits for longevity, including reducing the risk of heart disease, stroke, and diabetes, as well as improving mental health and cognitive function.

Resistance training, also known as strength training, is a type of exercise that involves exerting force against an external resistance (such as weights, resistance bands, or one's body weight) to build and tone muscle. This form of exercise is essential for preserving muscle mass and bone density as we age, as well as for enhancing physical function and mobility.

Flexibility and balance exercises, such as yoga and tai chi, increase joint mobility, balance, and coordination. These activities are particularly beneficial in reducing the risk of falls and improving general physical function in the elderly. They've also been linked to good psychological impacts including reduced stress and anxiety.

Including all three types of exercise in one's regimen may give a comprehensive approach to boosting lifespan and general health. It is crucial to highlight, however, that exercise frequency, duration, and intensity should be customized to an individual's age, fitness level, and general health state.

Exercise has been demonstrated to improve physical, mental, and emotional health, as well as lengthen life. We may enhance our physical, mental, and emotional health and live a longer, healthier life by including exercise in our everyday lives.

5.4. Creating an Individualized Workout Program to Promote Healthspan

Now that we understand why exercise is essential

and what types of exercise might help us live longer lives, the next step is to design an exercise program that is unique to each of us.

Before starting an exercise program, it is important to assess our current fitness level and health status, whether via a conventional medical checkup, a talk with a healthcare practitioner, or the use of fitness apps and wearable technologies.

To enhance our health and fitness, we must first analyze where we are and then devise a strategy that takes into consideration our specific requirements and objectives, right down to the exercises, frequency, and duration.

Aerobic activity, strength training, flexibility and balance training, and other activities should all be incorporated in a personalized exercise plan for longevity, with the precise exercises chosen for each individual depending on their preferences, fitness goals, and present health.

Working out with a partner, tracking our progress with fitness apps and wearable technology, and rewarding ourselves when we meet certain targets may all help us stay in our exercise routine and retain our motivation and consistency.

Lastly, being motivated and persistent with our strategy via different tactics will assist us in reaping the most advantages for a better and longer life. To summarise, building a personalized exercise plan for longevity requires a comprehensive evaluation of our present fitness level and health state, realistic goal setting, and the inclusion of various forms of exercise.

5.5. Physical Exercise and Its Role in Everyday Life

Incorporating physical activity into daily routines is an effective strategy to improve overall physical fitness, maintain healthy body weight, and reduce the risk of chronic diseases; this is why it is important to view physical activity as a lifestyle choice that includes regular physical activity throughout the day, not just as something was done during dedicated exercise sessions.

It is important to start with small, manageable goals and gradually increase the frequency and intensity of physical activity over time to reap the long-term benefits of exercise. Walking, cycling, gardening, and household chores are just a few examples of everyday activities that can help achieve the recommended amount of physical activity.

Prolonged sitting has been linked to an increased risk of cardiovascular disease, diabetes, and obesity; taking frequent breaks from sitting and engaging in light physical activity, such as stretching, walking, or standing, is an effective strategy for combating these negative health effects.

Choosing activities that are enjoyable and sustainable over the long-term, in order to maintain motivation and adherence to the exercise routine, is essential. Some examples of incorporating physical activity into daily routines include taking the stairs instead of the elevator, parking the car further away from the entrance, and walking to work.

Physical activity has been associated to gains in mental health, including fewer symptoms of anxiety and depression, and a lower chance of acquiring chronic conditions like cardiovascular disease, type 2 diabetes, and several types of cancer.

One study monitored approximately 1,500 persons over a 20-year period and showed that those who were physically active had a 35% lower risk of acquiring dementia compared to those who were sedentary. This finding applies to both Alzheimer's disease and other kinds of dementia.

According to another study, regular exercise can improve immune system function. Participants in the study regularly engaged in moderate-intensity exercise for 12 weeks, and by the end of the study, the participants' blood had a significantly higher concentration of immune cells than at the study's onset.

A study published in Cell Metabolism found that regular exercise can increase the production of a protein called SIRT3, which is involved in cellular metabolism and energy production and is associated with a reduced risk of age-related diseases such as type 2 diabetes and cardiovascular disease.

Integrating regular exercise into daily routines, along with other healthy lifestyle behaviors like a balanced diet, can help individuals maintain good health and well-being throughout their lives, as suggested by scientific data.

Group exercise classes, team sports, and outdoor recreational activities are just a few examples of physical activities that can be used as an outlet for socialization while also promoting physical activity and over all health.

In conclusion, physical exercise should be seen as a

way of life rather than a chore, with the prescribed quantity of physical activity being achieved through incorporating physical activity into daily routines, selecting fun and sustainable activities, and socializing through physical activity.

5.6. Conclusion

In this chapter, we discussed how exercise and physical activity can help you live longer by improving your physical health, mental health, cognitive function, and immune system. Exercise has been shown to reduce the risk of chronic diseases like heart disease, diabetes, and cancer, and it can even reverse some of the effects of aging.

Aerobic exercise, resistance training, and flexibility and balance training all provide unique benefits for longevity; therefore, it is important to incorporate a variety of exercises into our daily routines. Furthermore, it is crucial to create a personalized exercise plan based on individual fitness level, health status, and realistic goals to achieve the best results.

Making physical activity a habit and incorporating it into everyday routines can make it easier to maintain a consistent exercise plan, and interacting while engaging in physical activity can bring extra advantages for mental health and overall well-being.

To sum up, emphasizing physical activity in daily life is vital for sustaining optimal health and longevity, and we can all take steps towards a happier, more satisfying life by committing to regular exercise and incorporating physical activity into our daily routines.

CHAPTER 6: ENHANCING YOUR MIND: STRATEGIES FOR BRAIN HEALTH AND LONGEVITY

When we set out on our journey to investigate the complicated processes that take place in our brains, it is essential that we keep in mind the enormous breadth and depth of those processes. Even though the human brain is the most complex machine ever devised, there is still a great deal about it that scientists do not fully understand.

Even from the moment we are born, our brains are already evolving and becoming more complex. When we have new experiences, the neurons in our brain link with one another and rewire themselves, which results in the formation of neural pathways that influence our thoughts, feelings, and behaviors. These brain pathways serve as the basis for our memories, and they also make it possible for us to acquire new abilities and adjust to different circumstances.

On the other hand, as we become older, our brains lose some of their capacity to form and keep these neural networks intact. This decline is associated with an increased chance of acquiring neurodegenerative disorders as well as cognitive decline and memory loss. Yet there is no need to be concerned because there are techniques to improve brain health and increase longevity.

In this chapter, we will look into the most recent findings from scientific studies on how to keep your brain healthy and live a long life. We are going to delve into the complexities of our brains and figure out how to keep them healthy and functioning properly with some rather straightforward adjustments to our lifestyles. So, let's get started on this voyage of discovery together, where we will uncover the mysteries of the mind and figure out how to improve our mental capabilities so that we can enjoy a higher standard of living.

There is little doubt that the human brain is both intriguing and complex. It is frequently referred to as the "command centre" of the human body. It controls everything, from our bodily actions to our feelings, ideas, and behaviors, and it even controls our thinking. Yet, as we get older, different changes take place in our brains that have the potential to influence their function and structure. This can result in a decline in cognitive ability as well as memory loss.

Despite these shifts, research has revealed that there are a variety of approaches to maintaining optimal brain health and performance far into our senior years. We may improve brain health and longevity by adopting a healthy lifestyle, engaging in activities that stimulate our minds and our social relationships, and keeping up with the most recent findings from scientific studies.

As we progress through this chapter, we will investigate the most recent findings from scientific research on the relationship between brain health and longevity, discuss concrete strategies for improving brain function, and emphasize the significance of placing an emphasis on brain health as part of an all-encompassing strategy for healthy aging. Prepare therefore to challenge your cognitive abilities and discover novel approaches to extending the lifespan of your brain.

6.1. Methods for Improving Brain Health and Extending the Human Lifespan

a. Diet

The food that we eat not only contributes to the upkeep of a healthy body but also to the upkeep of a healthy brain and to the length of time that we can live. The nutrients that are required for healthy brain function can be supplied to the body by eating a diet that is both well-balanced and abundant in nutrients. It is possible to protect the brain from oxidative stress and inflammation, both of which are connected with cognitive decline and neurodegenerative illnesses, by eating foods that are rich in antioxidants, healthy fats, and foods that are anti-inflammatory.

Antioxidants, which can be found in fruits, vegetables, and grains that have been unprocessed, fight off dangerous free radicals that may cause cell death in the brain. It has been demonstrated that omega-3 fatty acids boost cognitive function and lower the risk of cognitive decline, making them a crucial component for maintaining brain health. These fatty acids can be found in fatty fish, nuts, and seeds. On the other hand, consuming a diet that is heavy in saturated and trans fats, sugar, and processed foods can lead to increased inflammation and oxidative stress, both of which can cause damage to the brain and cognitive impairment.

b. Exercise

Frequent physical activity provides a wide range of positive effects on health, including enhancements to cognitive performance and increased neuroplasticity. The creation of new brain cells and an improvement in cognitive performance are both outcomes of increased blood flow and oxygenation to the brain, which are brought about by physical activity. Also, it lowers the likelihood of developing neurodegenerative disorders as well as cognitive deterioration. Studies have indicated that maintaining a regular exercise routine can even reverse some of the impairments in brain function that are associated with aging.

c. Sleep

Sleep is critical to maintaining a healthy brain and proper cognitive function. During sleep, the brain can strengthen memories, cleanse itself of harmful pollutants, and replenish its supply of energy. There is a correlation between not getting enough sleep regularly and cognitive impairment, as well as an increased risk of neurodegenerative illnesses. The preservation of both brain health and cognitive function needs to get a sufficient amount of sleep each night.

6.2. Mental Stimulation and Social Engagement

a. Mental Stimulation

The ability to keep one's brain healthy and to live a long life are both dependent on one's level of mental stimulation. Improving cognitive function and lowering the risk of cognitive decline can be accomplished by participating in mentally taxing activities such as reading, solving puzzles, or acquiring new skills. The formation of new brain cells and the consolidation of existing neural connections are both facilitated by mental activity. According to a number of studies, engaging in mentally taxing pursuits can even put off the beginning of dementia.

b. Social Engagement

Participation in meaningful social activities is also essential to maintaining a healthy brain and a long life. Engaging in social interaction with other people is beneficial for mental stimulation, alleviating stress and depression, and providing a sense of purpose and belonging in one's community. On the other hand, research has shown that a deterioration in cognitive function as well as an increased risk of neurodegenerative illnesses is associated with social isolation and loneliness. Volunteering one's time or becoming a member of a group are two examples of social activities that might help improve cognitive performance and increase brain health.

6.3. Scientific Advances in Brain Health and Longevity

a. Brain-Computer Interfaces

Brain-computer interfaces, often known as BCIs, are devices that allow for direct communication to take place between a human brain and a computer. These interfaces circumvent the use of traditional channels, such as nerves and muscles. There is a possibility that BCIs will usher in a new era in the treatment of neurological illnesses and the improvement of brain function. In recent years, there has been significant progress made in the development of BCIs, which have been used to restore lost sensory and motor function as well as improve cognitive abilities such as memory and attention. BCIs have also been used to help people with conditions such as Parkinson's disease and multiple sclerosis.

The creation of brain prosthetics, which are devices that replace or enhance missing or injured sensory and motor function, is one of the most promising areas of research for BCIs. By converting a patient's brain signals into commands for a robotic arm or leg, for instance, a brain-computer interface (BCI) can help paralyzed patients regain the ability to move their limbs. In a similar manner, brain-computer interfaces (BCIs) have been utilized to give those who are blind the ability to "see" by transforming visual information into electrical impulses that are then sent directly to the brain.

In addition to regaining lost function, brain-computer interfaces (BCIs) may also be able to improve brain function in otherwise healthy people.

For instance, researchers are investigating the use of brain-computer interfaces (BCIs) to enhance memory and attention in patients suffering from traumatic brain injuries or cognitive disabilities. BCIs have the potential to improve cognitive function by stimulating specific parts of the brain with electrical or magnetic signals. This can increase neuroplasticity and stimulate the creation of new neural connections, both of which can lead to increased brain activity.

b. The neuroplasticity of the brain

The capacity of the brain to adapt and change in response to novel experiences is referred to as neuroplasticity. Recent studies have revealed that neuroplasticity can be manipulated to enhance brain function and increase the likelihood of living a longer life. Neuroplasticity is a process that continues throughout an individual's lifetime and can be strengthened through a variety of interventions including cognitive training, physical exercise, and stimulation of the brain.

Transcranial magnetic stimulation is one method that has shown some promise for improving the neuroplasticity of the brain (TMS). A non-invasive method of brain stimulation known as transcranial magnetic stimulation (TMS) employs magnetic pulses to target particular areas of the brain. TMS has the potential to improve cognitive function by targeting particular regions of the brain. This has the effect of enhancing neuroplasticity and promoting the creation of new neural connections in the brain.

Participating in mentally taxing activities like crossword puzzles, games, or learning a new language is an example of one method of cognitive training, which is another method for improving neuroplasticity. It has been demonstrated that cognitive training can both increase cognitive performance and lessen the likelihood of cognitive decline. Through presenting the brain with novel and difficult challenges, cognitive training encourages the creation of new neural connections as well as the strengthening of existing connections, which ultimately leads to an improvement in cognitive performance.

6.4. The Last Thoughts

In conclusion, maintaining a healthy brain is critical for living a long life and having a high quality of life. A healthy lifestyle, mental stimulation, and active participation in social activities are all effective methods for promoting brain health. New avenues of investigation in the fields of brain-computer interfaces and neuroplasticity have opened up exciting prospects for improving brain function and extending the human lifespan. We can keep our brains in peak condition and live lives that are rich in purpose and fulfillment if we implement the aforementioned tactics and keep up with the most recent findings in the scientific community.

7. THE FINAL THOUGHTS

"Inner Longevity: The Science and Art of Living Well for Longer" has explored the latest scientific discoveries and practical strategies for achieving optimal health and wellness, and living a long, fulfilling life. We are now aware of the latest findings in the study of ageing as well as the veracity of claims made for various anti-aging remedies. We have also explored methods for maintaining a healthy body and mind through things like diet, exercise, and mental stimulation. We learned firsthand that a few simple adjustments to our daily routine can have a significant impact on our health and happiness. The central idea of this book is that we have control over our own health and longevity. A life full of vitality, energy, and purpose can be cultivated through a preventative and holistic approach to health, as reflected in deliberate decisions regarding diet, exercise, and self-care. Let us, then, always keep our health as our top priority and work to improve it in any way we can. Let us seize the day and work together to build a better tomorrow. I appreciate you coming along with me on this adventure. Best of luck to you on your quest for true immortality.